SHIZOPHRENIA

DR. AFSAR M. SULAIMAN, QEP, REM

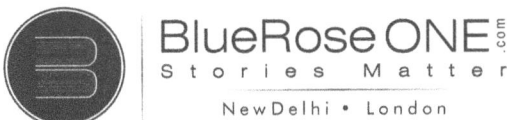

BLUEROSE PUBLISHERS
India | U.K.

Copyright © Dr Afsar M Sulaiman, QEP, REM 2025

All rights reserved by author. No part of this publication may be reproduced, stored in a retrieval system or transmitted in any form or by any means, electronic, mechanical, photocopying, recording or otherwise, without the prior permission of the author. Although every precaution has been taken to verify the accuracy of the information contained herein, the publisher assumes no responsibility for any errors or omissions. No liability is assumed for damages that may result from the use of information contained within.

BlueRose Publishers takes no responsibility for any damages, losses, or liabilities that may arise from the use or misuse of the information, products, or services provided in this publication.

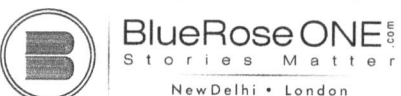

For permissions requests or inquiries regarding this publication,
please contact:

BLUEROSE PUBLISHERS
www.BlueRoseONE.com
info@bluerosepublishers.com
+91 8882 898 898
+4407342408967

ISBN: 978-93-7018-745-0

Cover design: Yash Singhal
Typesetting: Namrata Saini

First Edition: April 2025

Dedication

Dedicated to my offsprings who somehow consider me to be a schizophrenic!!!

Table of Contents

Schizophrenia: An Overview 1

Chapter 1: ECHO: voices poured in to the ears of supposedly a schizophrenic patient 3

Chapter 2: Comments' Redress: Voices' Interpretation 7

Chapter 3: Early Symptoms 11

Chapter 4: Universitylife: Worsening of Symptoms 16

Chapter 5: My Schizophrenic Professional Career 30

Chapter 6: Journey from Environmental Scientist to Environmemntal Writer 58

Chapter 7: Chronic Consequences of Shizophrenia 59

Chapter 8: Confession of Being Schizophrenic 61

Chapter 9: Epilogue 63

References/ Publications 65

About the Author 67

Schizophrenia: An Overview

Schizophrenia is a serious mental health condition that affects how people think, feel and behave. It may result in a mix of hallucinations, delusions, and disorganized thinking and behavior. Hallucinations involve seeing things or hearing voices that aren't observed by others. Delusions involve firm beliefs about things that are not true. People with schizophrenia can seem to lose touch with reality, which can make daily living very hard.

People with schizophrenia need lifelong treatment. This includes medicine, talk therapy and help in learning how to manage daily life activities.

Because many people with schizophrenia don't know they have a mental health condition and may not believe they need treatment, many research studies have examined the results of untreated psychosis. People who have psychosis that is not treated often have more-severe symptoms, more stays in a hospital, poorer thinking and processing skills and social outcomes, injuries, and even death. On the other hand, early treatment often helps control symptoms before serious complications arise, making the long-term outlook better.

(MAYO CLINIC)

Following chapters discuss a case history, for professionals and specialists in the arena to conclude if the case is the case of Schizophrenia?

CHAPTER 1

ECHO: voices poured in to the ears of supposedly a schizophrenic patient

You need to see a good doctor for your mental health, you are shameless, your supplications are show off, you are not what you pretend to be, you bring shame and disgrace to everyone you come in contact, I will burn everyone and the dwelling if your actions led to any mishap, I think you should consult a good doctor and ask if you have Schizophrenia, your father was a womanizer and a drunkard, who does not know that, it was because of him that your mother lost her senses, unfortunately the same blood flows in our veins, we as children always tried to save grace and showed you in the best of light to everyone (WHO? Nanihal, Dadihal, Friends like having office in Meridian???or Sasural??) But you are showing your true character through your filthy write up (not a book of any standard) (in front of who?? You type of highly qualified and experienced literature wizards ???)) has destroyed it all, you are a selfish man (requires an honest introspection by each one of you>>???), (except two in a limited sports arena, what grace you brought and think you have impacted your relatives far and wide with your performances??? Except showing of what you have and can do with money and stating I can eat what I want, wear what we want and travel whereever we wish???) you want everyone to die before you (a timid statement of a fearful baby who has not grown up well emotionally) and don't want your children to live gracefully but shamefully throughout their remaining lives, you have been an unfaithful husband to all your wives like your father and an unfaithul father, whatever you have written is your point of view....others have theirs too, the famous lines you quote that aulad are a fitna (test), if you evaluate well, will understand it is otherway round,you are scared to talk because you cannot defend your lies (lies or opacity and translucency to all opaque and translucent highly acclaimed personalities of my household??), you have written bad for everyone who came close to you, be it all your wives...or anyone who had a bit affection(Oh really??? How much do you know???..........), whatever you have written is your point of view.....others also have...., this book will bring disgrace to you, (Review comments by Offsprings on my book MIRAGE, published recently), if something happens to me, don't come in my funeral, I don't want to have any relationship with you and so on and so forth....... You did not take our mother along on business trips far and wide for your enjoyment (ayyashi(, an statement by that son who had seen me closely abroad from 1985 to to 2002 ad afterwards as well, knowing well that family status is not on business trips by company policies, particularly for expats??? I am happy for this matter all my offsprings are together and in unison. All this mixtupness happened when one of my sons hacked my account and shared with another and started deducing inference based on partial truth, an act which is criminal as per the law of the land, also somewhat by blocking them they had put something in my phone that they are continuously monitoring my banking activites and messaging system, even sending derogatory remarks to my contacts, even thretening them on my belh from my phone None of my offsprings consider their acts incorrect, illegal or immoral!!! I may be the worst creature on earth, yet they neither have the right to encroach my privacy, good or bad. I would have been happier if they would have reported to the cyber police instead.

These words are for:

Dr. Afsar M. Sulaiman, a Qualified Environmental Professional (QEP) from Pittsburgh, Registered Environmental Manager from Illinois, Environmental Scientist and an International Consultant, has recently published his books, Balance and Mirage and now publishing an essence of his professional journey expanding to almost four decades. The new book, HAZAR is my trade, which is practically a hand book, meant for Environmental Science and Engineering students, teachers and professionals.

He is an Alig who was enrolled in 1972 in PUC and completed his PhD in Environmental Chemistry in 1983 from the Department of Applied Chemistry, Z. H. College of Engineering & Technology, AMU, Aligarh. His career started from the IIT Bombay as a Research Scientist. He was responsible for the establishment of the first Environmental Management Company in the Middle East, National Environmental Preservation Co. Jubail, Saudi Arabia. During his four decades of services for environmental cause, he was awarded International Man of the Year was featured in Five Hundred Leaders of Influence, MARQUIS Who's Who in the World, Saudi Gazette in 1998-99. He presented his papers in several international conferences. He travelled the world to find the best environmental technologies, best suited for the Middle East in general and Saudi Arabia in particular. He has established several environmental companies, outfits and establishments across Saudi Arabia, Bahrain, Qatar and UAE. He has just last year published his first book BALANCE (Meezan) on Environmental Management in the light Holy Scriptures and traditions of the Prophet Mohammed PBUH, and another book MIRAGE, about his life (a sort of autobiography).

Whatever, written in Mirage is nothing but plain truth from my perspective of course, if no one can understand and read between the lines are their outlook, no one can help.

I am me and whatever I am, have proved, and known globally by hard work and the grace of the Creator. None of you can claim to add any feather in my cap.

CHAPTER 2

Comments' Redress: Voices' Interpretation

My father, a judge of British era, told me once how he started drinking. The toughest time upon him used to be when he had to pronounce a death sentence. He used to be in <u>schizophrenic</u> frame of mind before and after, pronouncing a death sentence. His one of the closest friends, Justice Jugal Kishore advised him to take a couple of pegs to ease his internal environment. He never was a drunkard as per accounts of all those who knew him well, including my elder siblings. My mother never ever disrespected him in anyway despite her huge age difference. She used to love him, cared for him when in senses. Yes, she used to be either self-destructive in depression and in an excitement phase she used to be violent, and hit my father with anything that used to come handy. Several times my fatter was hurt but never complained or said a word to her. When situation used to be out of control at home, she used to be admitted in the mental hospital in Kanke, Ranchi under care of a fatherly Dr Haseeb, who later became maternal father-in-law of my elder brother from my second mother.

My father was named a womanizer because he married thrice by my otherwise jealous relatives. My first mother died right after giving birth to my eldest brother, probably due to TB, an incurable disease those days.

He was married to my second mother, elder sister of my mother, upon been approached by my maternal grandfather, Professor Wahid-Ur Rahman, Head, Department of Physics, Osmania University , Hyderabad. My second mother died of probably Cholera after giving birth to her fourth child. My mother then only in teens started taking care of my second sister of 6 months.

My maternal grandfather, insisted my mother and father to get married. My father used to respect my maternal grandfather very much. My mother too used to adore her father, could not refuse and got married.

On second day of her marriage, my mother had the first attack of mental imbalance and started doing weird things like throwing her books out of the cabinet. She was the brightest student in her class and had to abandon her studies. During last days before independence of India. British Forces were rampant in their overtures particularly targeting Muslims. My maternal grandfather was so scared that he fled from Hyderabad to his native village with no facilities for girls' education. Having no other suitable choice for my mother then, he probably took the decision of my mother's marriage with my father.

The above is a truth as narrated by my father to me and even as narrated by my elder brothers and sisters.

No known facts or reference are existent for my father for being a womanizer or being responsible for my mother's mental health.

I do feel now that I am a schizophrenic person.as all my life, I tried to be impractically be like my father in most of my affairs. I am proud to be his son and up in heavens he is proud of me too.

I have been impulsive all my life probably, a rebel to so called traditions and pseudo idealism. What people think about me; I did not care right after becoming 21. My attitude gave me the best and the worst. I own all my deeds in full and consider myself responsible, no one else.

Timid personalities blame conditions to be responsible for being hindrance in their progress and successes. And supplicate to the One and Only

Hazar barq giray, lakh aandhiyan aayein,

Wo phool khil kay raheingay jo khilnay walay hain.

If anyone is a non- achiever, is because of his not trying to know difference between work and fatigue, his weakness of being non-directional, failing to fulfill his duties assigned (during studies wasting time and money and resources for personal enjoyment and overtures on free money not earned but received from someone's blood money), preference of rest and sleep during working hours, being out of focus, having no values for others money earned through hard work and considering that money as their rights......................!!!????

Yes, I am schizophrenic by descent too, my mother used to be admitted frequently in mental hospital!!!

I am like my father rather more than him by your definition of womanizer. He married thrice and I did four times. He never had affairs; I had. I am not a pseudo idealist and never will be. I am a real person, living in a real world not in Utopia. I do have common weaknesses and strengths of a normal being. If I feel, I did wrong do something good to lessen my sin and supplicate to the One and Only, admitting my weaknesses, it is no one's affair to talk about my relationship with my Creator as none know what that means ???!!!. (Essence of Hadith). Know before you speak else will make mockery of yourselves.

For me, marriage is an agreement (as per Islamic laws as well)or a contract. And could be annulled under certain conditions. It's not a Catholic marriage or even Hindu marriages. I can marry four at a time. If one is overpowered by his or her ignorance then Ignorance tax (IT) has to be paid.

Do you know what faithfulness means? It means compliance to one's commitment. One has to find out if I was compliant or not???!!!

As regards shamelessness, one has to define what shameless is and in light of what? Own concept? As per Islamic laws? International laws?

Except for personal perception, everyone is shameless to one degree or the other. When a husband show-cases his wife in public is shamelessness, takes his wife to mixed gathering is shamelessness, if he doesn't correct actions of his family is shamelessness, if one lies to parents is shamelessness, if sons deceive parents is shamelessness, if sons use his hard-earned money on overtures is also shamelessness by law as well which we all claim to be followers. Covering up and condoning major sins is shamelessness??? Being with and enjoying their company are not only shamelessness but being party to that as well. Spending money on someone is not respectfulness? It's mere show off charity to let others appreciate a son to be exemplary, nothing else (a schizophrenic perspective which is religious as well!!).

A person's real character and characteristics get exposed during anger and hunger (of anything). Sometimes I deliberately create a situation to know Who is Who???

By the grace of Almighty, I know myself with all my weaknesses and all associated with me very well. A few know, I am well trained in Behavioral Sciences and my ability and capability has been used internationally.

CHAPTER 3

Early Symptoms

The supposedly, a schizophrenic patient was sent with my elder brother from my second mother, elder sister of my mother, to Jammu, where he was posted as a doctor. I was admitted to a Nun Convent School. The school considered to be the best in the region but a cultural shock for me. It took a while to adapt to altogether different environment. Initially, my English was too bad and was supposed to speak in English. One day due to some reason, I was absent from the class. When the next day I was asked for the reason, I somewhat responded , 'rain was falling jhama jhum, fisal gaya leg aur gir gaye hum, iss liye ma'am I could not come'. The whole class burst into laughter. I felt humiliated and started hating my school. My brother was very strict with me, more than my father. He used to scold me quite often and slap mercilessly for small mistakes and not doing so well in the class. He never cared about my likes and dislikes. He used to call me Zooria (a liar). He used to make me feel by his actions, that I was not his brother but someone forced upon him to take care of. My both parents used to give him utmost importance. I literally became his slave and a meek boy with no confidence. I met a sweet girl Nayana, who used to be quite sympathetic to me and sit beside me to soothe me and little bit teach me spoken English. A very natural bond was formed between us. In a few months, my brother resigned to join as a doctor in NCDC, Pathakhera, in Betul, MP. The hut colony was in the middle of the forest. I was forced to go once again with my elder brother for schooling. It used to be a nightmare. Nothing used to be there, no sign of civility, school or recreation. I cannot forget this incidence ever that once I saw a large bar of Cadbury Milk Chocolate in his cabinet without doors. I was too tempted and ate half of the bar First time in my life I was beaten by his chappal.

There were only two girls in the colony Bubbly and Sonia, sisters ,daughters of the General Manager, Mr. Rai. Both parents of the girls were very sweet and caring. They were the only children to talk to and play with. Here both sisters taught me how to kiss and hug. I was sent to a boarding school, Bishop Cotton School, Nagpur, Maharashtra. I was put in a boarding, All Saints House, for senior girls and primary boys. Jean, Joan and sister Lisa used to hug and kiss me a lot. I became their toy to play with. They used to enjoy my company a lot. They were kind and very affectionate. I was admitted to Standard II, was promoted to Class III in a month. In three months, I was promoted to Standard IV. I was doing quite well in the class and in extra-curricular activities. Once, Mr. and Mrs. Rai were on official visit to Nagpur and brought for me several large packets of biscuits. It was more feast for June who used to persuade me for those biscuits. The day I cleared exams, a bomb shell hit me badly. My brother resigned to join IOC, Refinery Hospital Barauni, built on our ancestral land. Our father persuaded him to take up this job so that he could be near to his family. Once again, I was back home and wanted to stay with my parents. I gave reasons to my mother why I did not want to go to live with my brother. She probably said something to him. He was very much infuriated and asked me sternly to follow him to Borhna Bari, a piece of brick walled land used for growing vegetables. I was barely 10 years then. He started scolding me with words I don't remember well but were humiliating and intimidating. His slave, me, could not muster strength to say anything. He started telling me how much of his money I had wasted while in schools and threatened me to show accounts of my expenditure to our parents while I was with him. My hate for him deepened. I was sent to the Public School, Darbhanga. Here I met a chubby girl, Vina, who used to share the class bench with me. She had very sweet demeanor. She used to share her delicious tiffin with me and became my dance partner in dance classes. She used to adore me and used to often say, I like you too much. She was very possessive. Never liked me to talk to other girls. After final exams, I went home and insisted my parents to put me in a local school and I joined a local school in Bihat a kilometer and half from our home. Another cultural and linguistic shock was awaiting. The medium of instruction was Hindi I did not know much, books were in Hindi and on top of it, by knowing, I am so poor in Hindi, comments of twenty monster type, girl classmates, and their teasing, living in India and unaware of Hindi (Bharat mein rahtay hain aur Hindi nahi aati !!! hahaha). This made me to concentrate only on Hindi and in six months started participating in all school events of debates, speeches and like on subjects of not my interest at all such as Tulsi Jayanti, Ram Charitra Manas and like and started bagging first prizes. My Hindi was forced amalgamated with Sanskrit vocabulary. Sanskrit dictums were forced into my debates and speeches. One of those I still remember,

Jawat jiwet sukhang jiwet, rinang kirtwa ghirtang piwet (Till you live, live merrily even take loan and drink ghee. In other words, 'Eat, Drink and be merry'). I cannot forget my innocent dear friend and classmate, Nehal from a nearby village, Rupaspur, who taught me how to ride a bicycle. I used to ride scissor style. He told me that he would teach me how to ride a bicycle properly. He said he was holding the back and asked me to mount on the seat of it. He said pedal. I did , and started pedaling. I was riding very well and found, he never was holding the back. He was developing my confidence. He was drowned dead during Ganges floods. I was devastated. Now even monster girls were keen to befriend and some even wrote love letters. My teachers loved me a lot and made me physical education lead of the school. My English speeches, particularly made all now sorry for their attitude towards me. I stood second in the class.

Next year was Standard VII, which was supposed to be a Board Examination. My determination became very strong to top and then, I became somewhat,

Hamein duniya say kya matlab, kutubkhana watan mera,

Mareingay hum kitaboun pay, waraq hoga kafan mera.

(What have I to do with the world? Library is my country, Will die on books and pages will be my shroud).

I topped the region but that year Seventh Board was dissolved.

I topped Class VIII and in IX. In the middle of the session of IX, a Punjabi girl, Anita Sayal, joined the class. A sweet girl in Shalwar suit with muffler type dupatta, with lower gaze and the only chashmish (spectacled) girl in the class. My Urdu and Persian classes used to be conducted in the other room because of fewer numbers of such students. While walking in the corridor, she started walking with me as if going in the same direction. She meekly said, keeping her gaze down, 'Will you please share your notes, I have to catch up with the class'. Her request was so genuine, I could not refuse, although my notes used to be jealously guarded property. When my notes were returned, was accompanied with a Thank You note and bouquet of words of admiration, her liking for me and beyond. I was somewhat clean bowled. Exchange of letters continued for months and final exam approached, I topped the class again. In Standard X, exchange of letters continued in its more colorful and poetic fervor. I met her only once in her backyard in front of my closest friend Deepak Sharma. We both remained mum during our encounter as both could not speak to each other and I left. Then came the Board Examination, all became busy. Right after the examination, my closest school friend Deepak Sharma, a Punjabi, informed that her father has been transferred to Bhakra Nangal and they are leaving tonight. Sky had fallen upon me. It was the darkest night, ever. I rode all the way to the Barauni Junction on my bicycle to see them off and she left my life, forever. I received a letter for stopping communication and to concentrate on studies.

My mother, often used to say,

'Puranay khatoun ko jala do, warna wo tumhein jala deingay' (Burn old letters otherwise they will burn you).

I showed all those letters to flame.

I topped the region in the High School.

CHAPTER 4

Universitylife: Worsening of Symptoms

After the High School, applied for admissions to various colleges including the Aligarh Muslim University. Got intimations from Saint Xaviers, Ranchi, Saint Columbus Hazaribagh, Patna Science College. I was intending to join the Patna Science College due to nearness from my parents. When I decided, the same night, after Tahajjud, my mother came to my room and made me take oath that I would take admission at the AMU, nowhere else.

Dates of admissions for above colleges, expired. Abba was furious for my inaction. I was rebuked like anything. In the first two lists of the AMU admission , my name was not there, I was deep inside scared to death. After 15 days, in the third and the last list, my name appeared in the last. My respect for Abba increased that day very, very much because whenever in earlier classes, I used to top, he never praised me rather used to say, Mian yahan andhoun mein kana raja ho, dekheingay jab tum rajaoun mein raja banogay (You are here, one eyed king among blinds, will see if you could become king among kings). Hearing such words used to be painful but the day I found my name at the end of the last -list, I realized prophecy of my father's words. He made me understand where really did I stand in a national scenario.

To cut short, I landed at the AMU on 04 August 1972 with a trunk and a hold all on a cycle rickshaw through Bab Ur Rahmat in Sir Syed Hall to my cousin Afroz Rabbani's room, who was managing my admission. I got a four seated room in Sadr Yaar Jang Hostel (B Block), Ross Masood Hall.

The first day of the PUC class was simply exhilarating as my teachers were simply too good in teaching and their affectionate demeanor. Dr. Afridi of Botany, Dr. Mashhood of Chemistry, Dr. Farhan Mujeeb of Physics, Dr. Athar Siddiqui of Zoology, all of them very good and stylish orators. I was on the seventh sky realizing that I have been blessed with teachers I craved for furthering my career in Medicine, a wish of my father to see me as a doctor.

I did start my studies with all zeal and enthusiasm but Aligarh's all Ms. (Makhi, Machchar, Matri, Makkhan etc.) became somehow my rivals. I spent most of my time in the University Health Centre for Malaria and typhoid. I appeared in my PUC examination and got sixth position in the university with distinction in three subjects, thank to my sincerity in High School studies when I used to refer higher level books.

Second year was Pre-medical (PMC). Despite rivalry with all Ms. and communal riots in the region and closure of university time to time, I put all my efforts and did fairly good in the PMC. It was a crucial time as I had to appear in the competitive tests. I appeared at the AMU, JIPMER Pondicherry, Maulana Azad Medical College, Delhi. I was in the waiting list in JIPMER, I was disqualified at Maulana Azad because my right eye was 6/60. At the AMU, my senior roommate, now a retired professor Dr. Mateenul Islam congratulated me for the selection. I was overjoyed and could not wait to reconfirm and went straight to my parents to break the news and get my uniform made. When I returned back for the admission, I saw my name in the waiting list at 11th place.

According to my seniors, it was some misappropriation in the list and that had happened. Anyway, I could not get the medical seat. Next session of B.Sc. II year I dropped for the preparation for the next year test and I did try my best but somehow that fire was lacking. I did appear in various tests but everywhere I was in the waiting list. I reluctantly joined B.Sc. Chemistry Honors II year.

This year something happened which never should have happened. I was invited by my classmate with nickname, Mickey for lunch at his home. There I met his family members including his younger sister Uroosa, aged almost my age. She was continuously gazing at me. I was quite uncomfortable. When my friend and others left for washing their hands for lunch, she directly said that she loved me and wanted to marry me. I was taken aback. I was simply speechless. When my friend and their mother returned, there was meaningful smiles on their faces. I suspected those moments of seclusion with Uroosa was deliberately given. A new tale of my life had begun. Uroosa often used to come at the gate of my hostel and used to summon for something important. Fearing what others would think, I used to meet her and go to cafes far away to hear her story of deep love for me. I got slowly involved and started longing for her. One finds morning, a hostel fellow, Afroz Taj, a poet and a great singer of our university knocked my room and said he got married to Uroosa the other day. I was speechless but managed to congratulate him. He was senior to me. Later came to know, Mickey was involved very closely to Afroz's sister who was probably pregnant. He married her and Afroz married to Uroosa. I was broken, yet diverted my attention by watching a lot of movies, smoking and getting dead tired, enough to drop dead in my bed. Fortunately, I did not ignore my classes and studies. It was final year of BSc, and I was walking through the lane of Morrison Court, a hostel, my nephew used to stay in. He saw me and came to me and questioned why I was still there. I was confused and asked what had happened. He informed my father expired 10 days ago. It was a bombshell impact. I hurriedly caught the first available train home. When I entered the main gate, my motherly elder sister, Rafiya Baji rushed to me and asked to restrain as Amma had lost her mental balance. After a day everyone forced me to go back and prepare for the examination. Nobody remembered if I needed anything. I returned without enough to buy even a meal of a rupee. Prayed for the divine help. I locked myself in my room. My dues were due without which Hall ticket could not be had. I was fearing of losing a year. First 24 hours passed without food, 48 hours passed, nothing happened, when 72 hours was about to finish, I heard a knock on my door. I was too weak to open, yet, somehow, I did, holding the door not to fell down. I saw my Jordanian classmate Hassan Abdulaziz Abdul Majeed Abdul Waheed. He told me that he would like to take tuitions in chemistry as all of his chemistry papers from the first year were uncleared. I thought he needs tuition as a classmate. As I was weak and I could only say okay but after tomorrow. He forced some notes into my pocket and left. It was enough to clear my dues and sustenance for a couple of months. Allah's help did come. I put all my energy to coach him and simultaneously I was getting revised and ready for the examination. Hassan passed all his chemistry papers fairly well and came to thank me for my diligence and said that now he can continue getting his scholarship. I was immensely happy that I am worth something. Hasan became my marketing help and informed all foreign students at AMU about me. There was an influx of foreign students for Chemistry and English, later Physics as well. I started sidewise international student tutoring in batches of Iranian boys, Iranian girls, Somali boys and girls, Iraqi boys, Palestinian boys etc. Every month I was making not less than a professor those days. My confidence was enhanced and started doing for family in a modest manner on both sides.

One of my batchmate, Zulfiqrul Islam Hashmi, Ahsan, from Commerce Stream, requested for teaching her elder sister, Rana, English during weekends as gesture of goodwill. After a week or so, he insisted for the dinner so insistingly, I could not decline. That day

I met his mother, Zahra Hashmi, a very graceful lady always ready to cook very pleasantly even for strangers. I was very impressed with her attitude and sincerity. Several dishes were served in the dinner but I could not take any as all of them were very hot except Arhar dal served in a crystal bowl of British era. It was so good that I could not resist to ask, who did prepare that. I was told his younger sister Farzana. I continued going on weekends at his place for tutoring Rana. Tea used to be very good at his place, prepared by Farzana/Farro.

Gradually Ahsan's mother developed a sort of motherly affinity with me and started sharing a lot of family affairs with me. During this period, I noticed that both parents of Ahsan were on different wavelengths of understanding and Farzana, a misfit in the periodic table. While mother wanted to live like others in the society, the father wanted to live within his means. This used to be the major apple of discord between the two. Farzana never went to school like rest of her siblings. She used to take care of household and her father particularly who was a heart patient. During conflicts, mother used to take all her children to her own parents to teach father a lesson in order to bend his ideals. Farzana never accompanied her mother rather took care of her father by cooking for him, making frequent tea for him, giving water in the washroom and like needs. One day, during her turbulent time she told me that she is worried about Farzana, as she was neither appropriately educated because of her non-interest nor she was otherwise abled as girls of those days. I was surprised yet continued to listen patiently and attentively in all obedience. She continued and said even she is ready to get her married with a peon. This made me very much pained and without thinking anything, I said, if you are so desperate, I am ready to marry her despite I have only given my B.Sc. examination. She looked at me with utter disbelief but apparently relieved.

I passed B.Sc. with first division and my name appeared in the list of Biochemistry for M.Sc. admissions. Although Biochemistry used to be considered the best those days, did not suit my side business for sustenance. The classes used to be continuously, from 7 am to 5 pm. Upon checking other options, found that in Analytical Chemistry classes conclude at 2 pm. I completed admission formalities for the Masters in the Analytical Chemistry without missing visit to Nai Basti where Asan's family lived in a rented house. On one weekend, when I knocked the door, Farzana opened the door, her face swollen, a face as it appears after long weeping. I was not ready for this but was shocked. I asked if everything was okay and she said all are at granny's place and I am alone. I apologized and left. That night was not normal for me. I was not able to sleep. Farzana's pained face was in my eyes. Just before morning prayers, I had decided.

The next morning, I appeared in the office of Mr. Miftahul Islam Hashmi , father of Farzana. He welcomed and asked to sit and asked the reason of my visit to him. Without any preface, I calmly said, I wanted to marry Farzana and needed his blessings. He was shocked and stood up with mixed emotions of anger and disbelief. He said, it is your study period, concentrate on that. Don't do anything that will compromise on your education for which you are in the university. I simply responded that I was not worth anything but would keep Farzana better than her current status and left. I was very light that day.

Probably Farzana's father broke the news of the day to his spouse. She took a stand on my behalf and declared to all relatives; Farzana is getting married to me. No one was happy among Farzana's relatives. Her maternal uncle was furious and asked who the hell Afsar was. Farzana's mother was rock determined and cared for none and on 10th November 1977,which happens to be my real Birthday also, afternoon, my Nikah was carried out in most simplistic manner after Asr prayers in three pairs of clothes brought by me. I simply gave mere a 50 rupee note for seeing my bride. No rituals, no gana bajana (singing and music) and I took my wife to the best hotel in the town those days, India Hotel. Both were amateur for the night.

Next morning, left for the so-called honeymoon to Delhi. Stayed at Hotel Naaz at Jama Masjid, Delhi. Making it the epicenter, started going to Farzana's Delhi relatives. Best memories remain of her Ehtesham Mamu and Ghazala Mumani. They were adorable and her cousin Fouzia/Fouzi. We returned in a few days back to my rented tiny house in Aligarh to start our new phase of life. Spending a few weeks with Farzana made me feel that she was a divine blessing for me. She proved that she was a bouquet of wife, mother, sister, daughter and a soulmate. I was happy with my decision despite angering my own kith and kin.

Anwar was so furious at my marriage that he not only blasted me mercilessly in his epistle to me, did too mean stuff. My Samiya khala, younger to Amma, forced left this world by burning herself. She left behind some jewelry. Two most learned persons and considered wisest, Anwar and Asghar those days decided to make a fund for needy in the family by selling them. Practically he became custodian of that fund. After my marriage, he withdrew some 9500 rupees from that fund against his expenditure on me to date and informed me in stern words to pay into the fund that amount.

It was marriage of my younger sister, Tayyaba, we bought some gifts and left for Nurpur to attend her marriage. Farro was in the family way. In order to avoid unpleasant situation, we checked into a hotel in Begusarai and went to our home. Knowing I had come, Anwar announced if I will attend the marriage he will not. Decision was in his favor and we could not attend the ceremony. After the ceremony, he came to pick us up to his place and blasted me like anything in front of Farro. To cut short, we were provided permit to enter the ancestral home. We went there and Amma embraced Farro saying, one daughter has left, another came in. Many multiples of that 9500 was given to deserving on behalf of the departed soul without informing anyone as I did not believe in that fund's legitimacy or legitimacy of the custodian.

Knowing that Farzana was never named as per Shariyah rituals, Aqeeqah, a goat was slaughtered and I named her Farhana Afsar against Islamic ethical code, should had been Farhana Saeed Hashmi, due to my ignorance. Farro remained Farro but.

I developed very strong bond with my father-in-law due to his character. He was a thorough gentleman with firm belief, attitude and sincerity. We became friends. We used to smoke together have tea together and used to have open and frank discussions. Gradually I came to know him very well. He used to support his colleagues financially as used to receive handsome amount from his father who used to be very much financially sound. Some of his colleagues retired as professors. Irony was when he himself joined AMU, he used to get remuneration less than what he used to receive from his father. He never complained and remained patient throughout his life. Started living his life within his means. His helping nature often brought wrath from his spouse. He was an honest person, never did take advantage of his position or power. He adored me more than his own sons. He gradually became epitome of my respect.

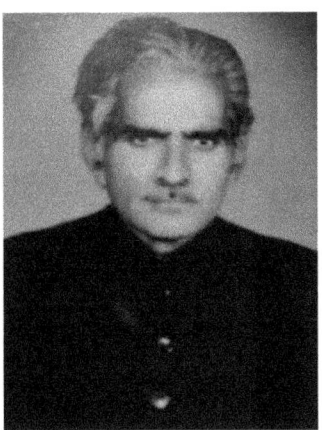

Miftah-ul-Islam Hashmi
My Father-in law

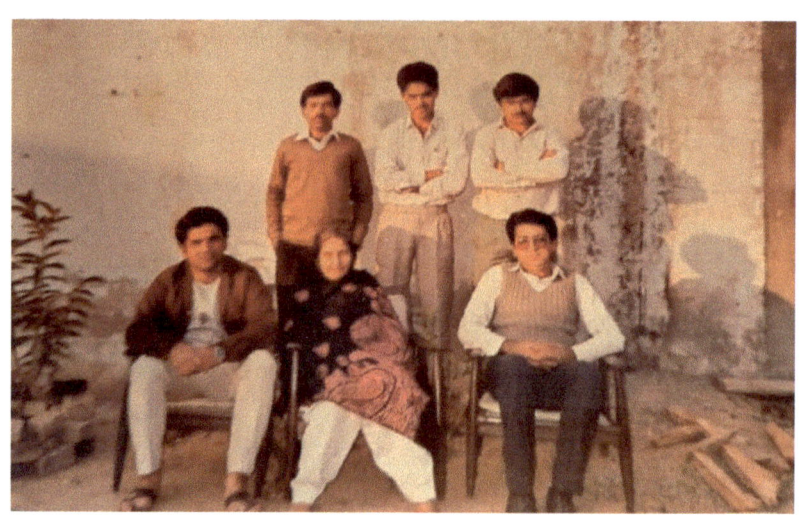

**My Mother-in-law with her five pillars
(Zehra Hashmi, Ahsan, Zia, Hashim, Shahid and Shamsi)**

Being still a student of the first year of M.Sc., I continued my classes and part time tuitions. She used to be alone yet very contended. I asked her to appear privately for the High School Examination from the AMU, Girl's School and started tutoring her in English and Hindi her weaker subjects. She cleared her exams and filled form for the PUC but got her first diploma named Saima. She was a joy for all particularly her Nanajan, who used to climb up the stairs just to read QUR'AN and blow her almost daily before going to his office. Once when I went to my hostel room, I found blood-stained intestines of probably goat or something on my doorstep. The moment I crossed it, I became sick, my heart started sinking and I managed to reach home somehow. He became so concerned, he started reading Qur'an on a glass of water and blowing both water and me for almost 45 minutes. He asked me to drink that Qur'an read water. Reluctantly I did. I was a bit better. The next morning, he took me to the Qazi of Aligarh, who was famed to be a spiritual healer, and requested him to do something. The Qazi saw my nails, eyes, smelled my hands and said I was victim of black magic. He read Qur'anic verses and blown my chest.

My restlessness eased and he asked me to read certain things from Quran after each salah (prayers). Then one day Rana became very serious and was hospitalized. No one offered to stay with her overnight in the hospital. Although I had my paper the next day, myself and Farro offered ourselves to be with Rana overnight to take care of her. It was biting January winter and there was no place in the General Ward to spread a sheet to straighten ourselves. We moved to the balcony and spent the whole night cling together in a blanket. The next morning Ammi came to the hospital with breakfast. I left for my examination. I did not do well as could not get time to revise the previous night. The city was gripped under communal violence and Papa had heart attack. We rushed him to the hospital but it was sine die. Hardly staff were there to take care. It was curfew all over. It was an ardent task to carry food to the hospital. We used to do so on a bicycle. Me, Farro and Ammi were only attendants. I took a hard decision to take Papa to AIIMS, Delhi. Only Ammi or any one attendant were allowed to be with the patient in the hospital. It was summer. I and Ammi were alternating. My second brother- in- law, Chummu (Ziaul Islam Hashmi) also accompanied us to Delhi. We used to straighten up on the pavement outside the hospital. On the third day, it was my turn to be with him. Suddenly Papa had another attack and lost his senses. Doctors tried everything but in vain. He had left for the heavenly abode. We brought him to Aligarh and he was laid to rest in Mintoi, the University Graveyard. It was hardest time for the family when we stayed with one of our relatives. Ahsan was given job on a junior level as per university policies. He became the only bread winner for the rest. He worked hard, gave private tuitions to meet both ends.

Then came the final year of my M.Sc., Dr Rawat was assigned as an Advisor for the Analytical batch. He had 600 marks at his disposal. He used to teach by writing on the black board. Everyone used to copy. I used to do the same. During first sessional test he gave me 16/20 while to others much higher marks. I could not resist and went to his chamber and asked, everyone had written from your notes only, where did I make mistake to get lower marks. He was very angry and asked me to leave as no one questions him. In the final year 600 marks, he crushed me to the extent, my students excelled over me. I lost all hopes of any scholarship to pursue my PhD. I started applying for jobs like sales representative, chemists and like. Where ever, I went for interviews, was told to pursue higher academics.

Fortunately, 4 Scholarships were announced for a project from The Department of Environment, New Delhi under Professor Mohsin Qureshi, Head Department of Applied Chemistry, Z. H. College of Engg. & Technology, AMU. I appeared for both written and oral tests and topped for the JRF.

I went to Delhi for an interview. Upon return, Rana too had left for the heavenly abode.

I started my PhD journey in December 1980, under Professor Mohsin Qureshi. On the first day when I visited him for the guidance to proceed, he asked me to write Abstracts of papers published on the subject, "On Field Detection and Semi-quantitative Determination of Air, Water and Soil Pollutants", the name of the project as well for last 10 years (1970-1980). I started sitting in library and seminar. After three months carrying four registers of Abstracts, I went to his office, while keep signing his administrative role, he said to do the same from 1960-1970 without raising his head. It was a signal to leave and do what was told to be done.

Now Farzana was supposed to appear for the PUC Examination but could not. She was blessed with another Diploma named Ahmad. She wanted now to do nothing but to take care of her two diplomas.

While I was pursuing the next level of the literature survey, a thought flashed in my mind and went back to my guide and said, if he did not mind, I would choose topic of my thesis and work accordingly. The topic, I proposed was, "Detection, Determination and Separation of Organic Pollutants containing Tertiary Nitrogen". I saw the first time, smile on his face. I furthered by asking his requirement for the award of PhD from his perspective. He replied, if I could publish a paper in journal of international repute, on detection, determination and separation each, I will fulfill his requirements. I commenced the laboratory works and was able to get my first paper published in Water Research, Pergamon Press, UK 1982. I got soon after my MPhil. I continued my experiments and got my second paper published the same year in Journal of Liquid Chromatography(JLC), USA and at the end of the same year my third and fourth papers appeared in JLC and Science Reporter, India. I completed my thesis and took to my guide at his place for his signature. He outrightly refused and said no one had completed PhD in less than 5-7 years and that I should help others under him to complete their work. I got infuriated and slammed five copies of my thesis on his dining table saying that I am leaving but deal with him appropriately.

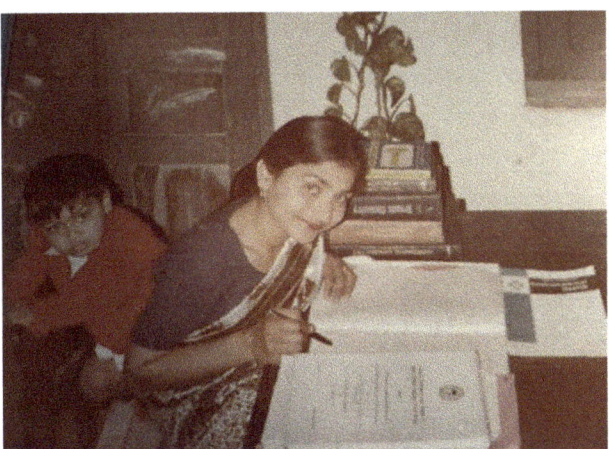

My Real PhD Guide

Next day I found my thesis with his signature. I hurriedly got them dispatched to the External Examiner in Hungary and IIT Bombay, Internal Examiner my guide himself and for archiving.

A month later both external examiners had sent their very positive reports. My guide had no choice than to submit his assessment as well. Examiner from the IIT, Bombay was supposed to conduct my viva-voce.

A few days later I had gone to the office to submit my contingency bills. I saw a letter from my guide to the IIT Bombay for delaying my viva voce for a year. I was aghast as my fellowship was ending after a couple of months. I rushed to Delhi and booked myself a chair car In Rajdhani Express for 150 rupees for Bombay Central. Next morning straight went to the office of my examiner, Prof. S. M. Khopkar, and introduced myself. I requested him to conduct my viva voce before leaving for Denver, USA as my fellowship was concluding soon and being a family man needed a job desperately. I also requested him not to inform my guide about my visit. He promised and kept it.

Next week he was in Aligarh and informed my guide that he was leaving for Denver for a year or more, thought to not delay my viva voce. I did very well in his grilling process. After it was concluded, he asked how could I do such an excellent work when there were not adequate facilities. I responded all due to supreme guidance of my guide and his gesture of goodwill. Second time, I saw smile on my guide's face.

I continued helping others in their works and simultaneously applying for jobs from Kashmir to Karnataka but no luck. At AMU, I was told by the Visitor's nominee, forget you will get job at the AMU. Son of my guide was selected. In Chandigarh, being a Muslim was the problem, In Karnataka, the interview was a mere formality, a person was already working and was confirmed for the position. Then came the call for interview for the position of Research Scientist at the IIT Bombay.

There were some 78 candidates for various positions for the same project, 'Bombay Environment Project'. At least 30 candidates were for the position I was supposed to be interviewed. I found myself weakest of the candidates in light of their knowledge, their eloquent English, their professional attitude and smartness. I prayed whether I am selected or not my university should not be defamed. It was the time of divine connection with the Almighty. I saw candidates entering and exiting in five minutes each. At the end I was called in. My interview continued for over an hour during which I was calm and composed and I don't remember a single question I did not answer appropriately. I was thankful that I did fairly well. I took Rajdhani back to Delhi and bus to Aligarh. Before I could speak a word, my wife handed over an Express Telegram informing me that I was selected for the position of the Research Scientist and should report for duties as soon as possible.

My both kids were in Our Lady of Fatima School, a good school indeed, I had to take them out, sold my household on whatever was offered and left with my family to Bombay to start my professional journey.

CHAPTER 5

My Schizophrenic Professional Career

It was altogether different set up and scenario. I was leading two JRF, an SRF and a Laboratory Assistant, a dedicated Jeep and a motor launch were provided for sampling and sea exploration. It used to be a thrilling job. My family often joined me on motor launch to Elephanta caves and sea survey of around Bombay - island.

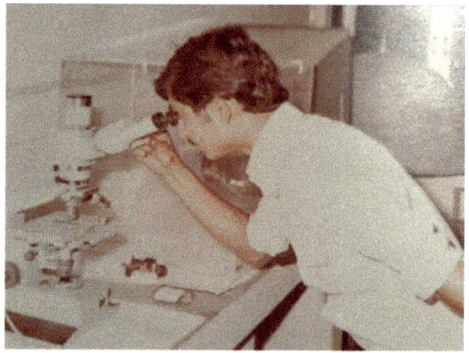

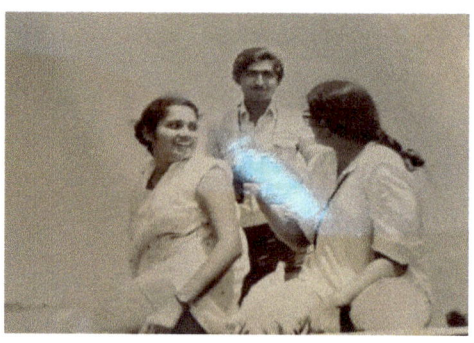

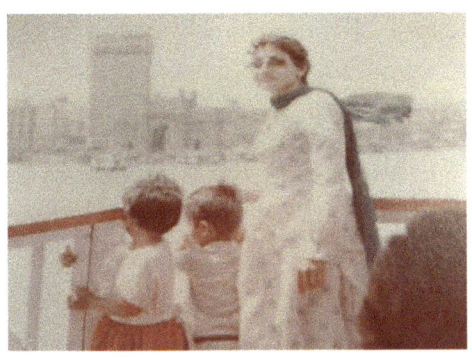

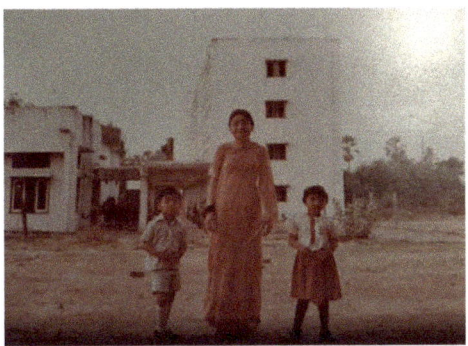

Glimpses of IIT Bombay

We were housed in a married hostel which was having a serene environment around. Hostel was having a canteen within. We used to mostly eat there as it was subsidized. Something, soon after a couple of months started bothering me. First education of my kids and the other regarding ethics of our leader. With my salary I couldn't afford schooling of my children and on the ethical front, the Project Manager started to instruct buying project requirements from specific suppliers. He used to give cash rebates. We were instructed to meet our travel needs and food from the same. Further my dream to help my mother and siblings were in dolls-drum. I started looking for the alternative. Then famous communal tensions grew in the region. My wife got scared as people started indecent commenting within IIT Campus. She started insisting to return back to Aligarh. Having little choice, without any intimation to my superiors, I took my family to my in-law's and returned back to join my duties. I was blasted like anything for uninformed travel. I could not take it and resigned impulsively.

Foreign recruitment was in progress as per ads in the newspaper. I sent my card to the Manager of the recruitment agency, CMC, Nariman point. I was allowed to meet the manager. I told him, I need a job desperately. He said if it was so, come for the written test the next day. If written test will be cleared, will be called for the interview. I cleared both and landed in Dammam, Saudi Arabia aboard Saudia. It was 16th June, 1984 and it was Ramadan. There were batch of 36 people joining the same organization, Saudi Kuwaiti Cement Manufacturing Co. (SAKUFA). We then boarded a bus, Ashok Leyland, which was without air conditioning system, to the work site, some 175 km deep in the desert region called Khursaniyah. It was a nightmare travelling through the desert at 48 degrees in the state of fasting of Ramadan. We were provided with porta cabins as accommodation and common toilets. Cabin was good enough for the two. We were supposed to be uniformed with safety outfits provided by the company. Food was provided free of charge and used to be very good. In three months, I was promoted to Supervisor and started leading 94 employees. My salary was doubled.

During this period, I visited my family once on my own expense and performed my first ever Umra. When I had reached Makkah Al Mukarramah, could not believe my eyes that I was there. I threw my luggage outside the entrance and rushed in to forget everything except eyes transfixed on Ka'aba. Tears streamed down and in the state of trans I started to talk to my Creator for how long I don't remember. It was Dohr's Adhan that made me to return to my senses. The Adhan itself simply caught my heart and I was overwhelmed. I started Umra ritual by Istelam and started Tawaf, an experience, cannot be worded. After the circumambulation, kissed Hajr-e Aswad, prayed at Multazim and offered two Rakah near Maqam-e Ibrahim, Wajib Ut tawaf, and proceeded to mount Safa to start Sai. After completion, got the hairs cut as per Qasar protocol. Umrah was completed. When I came out of Haram my bag was still there untouched. I changed and left for Jeddah to catch the flight to Madinah Al Munawwara. It was a very short flight. Checked into a hotel, 50 meters from the Haram. The keeper, a Pakistani Maulana type greeted with utmost affection and asked if I knew ethics of visiting Masjid-e- Nabawi Shareef. I simply sat beside him on the matted floor with inquisitive gesture. He affectionately and eloquently described each and everything. I was spell bound with his words loaded with love for Rasulullah Sallaho alaihi wasalam. I took shower, changed to white attire and wore itr and entered through Bab-e- Omar RA. Serenity descended upon me and I felt I am in Jannah. Performed two Rakah Tahayyatul Masjid and proceeded to the golden lattice to offer Salam. It was mesmerizing experience to be next to Nabi Kareem's final resting place. After offering salat o salaam, faced Ka'ba, under the silver domed window and made dua and offered Salam to Abu Bakr RA and Omar RA and exited the Masjid. Returned for Maghrib and Isha prayers. The next day was Friday. At Tahajjud Adhan, came to Masid e Nabawi and got a place in Reyazul Jannah, offered Tahayyatul Masjid and Tahajjud prayers. Then prayed at all pillars specially marked by Turkish architects, and at the Mimbar. Then read Qur'an on Ashab e Suffa platform and the platform next to the grill at the other end of the Rauza. Prayed Fajr, waited for Ishraq or Doha and returned to the hotel to catch up with sleep and prepare for Juma prayers. After Juma prayers, left for the airport to board flight to Dammam.

It was quite a divine journey to Holy Mosques and all I asked Allah were granted in just next couple of weeks. Alhamdulillah.

I was missing my family so badly that took a week without pay to be with them. Upon return was raised to Family Status and my family was with me in next couple months. We were provided with a three-bedroom luxurious villa with all hard and soft furnishings.

We had facility of subsidized meals catered by Oberoi caterings. Life was full of bliss.

It was late 1985, and my wife was in the family way, I was deputed as Superintendent, Quality Control at NABALCO, Australia and I had to leave within a week. I was reluctant to go due to my wife's condition. She insisted to go as doctors, nurses were available 24X7 within the precinct of the family campus, meals of all kind could be had on phone calls and by then she had befriended all ladies from India, Pakistan, Egypt, Jordan and Somalia due to her cooking skills and her sweet demeanor.

I left for Melbourne via Singapore, aboard Singapore Airlines. It was over eight hours direct flight. There was a layover of 24 hours. I booked a tourist bus ticket for sight-seeing. It was an experience right from the Changi Airport which in itself was a beautiful town with all one can think of. Travel by monorail and cable car were included. Variety of orchids in the botanical garden was quite fascinating. The cleanliness of the country was incomparable to most developed nations. Not a single cigarette butt, used tissue or spit sign could be seen anywhere, or even streets. People needing to spit, used to do so using tissue paper and dropping into trash bin nearby. I could see Islamic ethics of cleanliness everywhere and was very much impressed. Visiting to China town and India town were being in China and in India. I searched for an Indian vegetarian restaurant. I found a hut in traditional Indian village setting. I was told by Pundit ji to sit on a mat, spread over a clay floor. He brought a freshly washed banana leaf and kept in front of me and served four kinds of vegetables, dal, pickles, chapati and rice and was asked to start. During having this sumptuous meal, he continuously fanned me with a palm made fan.

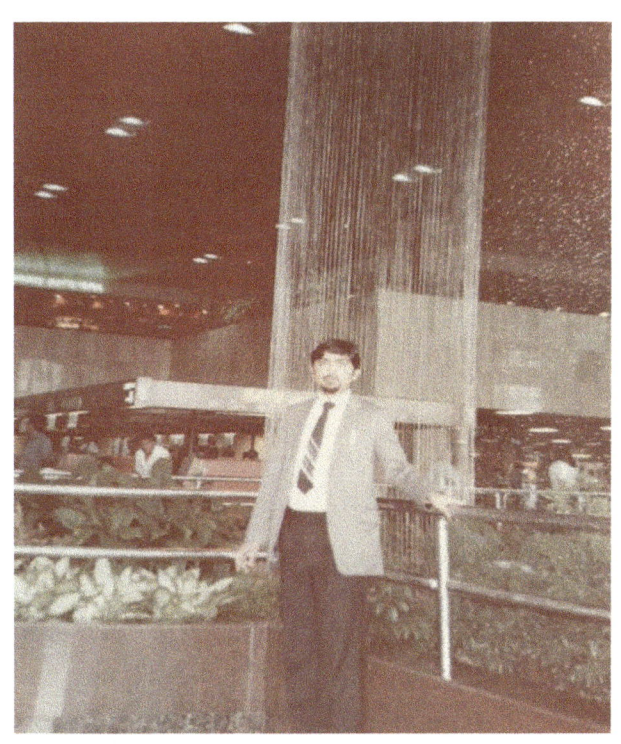

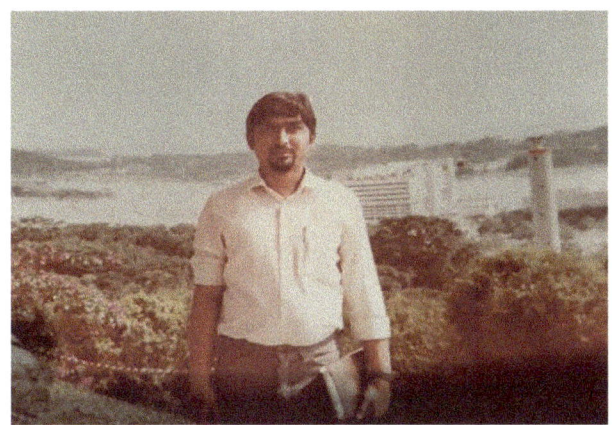

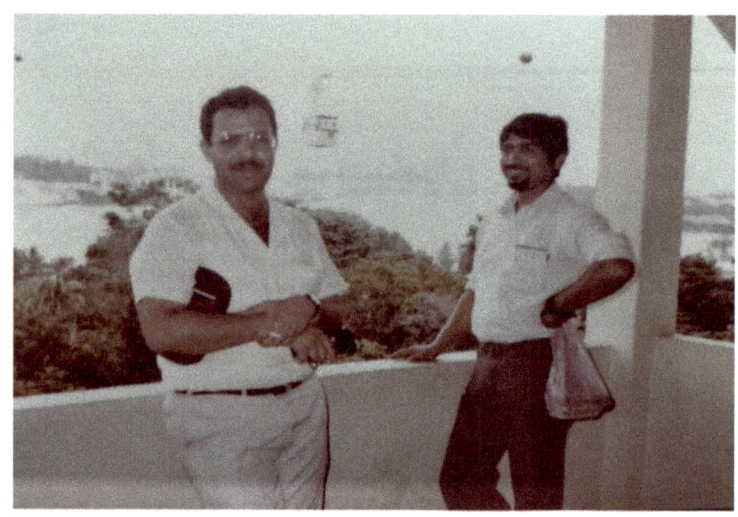

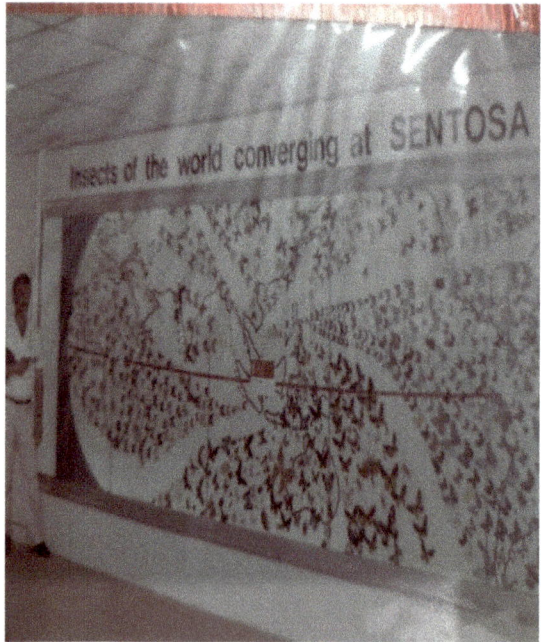

Glimpses of Singapore

The same night flew to Melbourne aboard, Quantas. It was again a flight over 8 hours. Lost sense of time while travelling to Southern hemisphere. When landed it was found to be summer.

Should have checked before the travel to avoid carrying weighty winter outfits.

Several meetings were conducted on yacht, cruise and 7-Star resorts. My first such an experience in life but instead of getting fascinated was uncomfortable throughout due to practices witnessed were against ethical standards I was raised with. There was flow of liquors of all kinds taken by both genders shamelessly. There was no ethics in vulgar touches of wives of others and that was rather norm than exception. A lady approached me seeing me sipping 7-UP. She asked if I was a man, as men take Cognac straight, whisky on rocks. I was unaware of such terminologies. I only said we prove manhood in private not public. This was probably a slap on her face and called me a rude. Anyway, the episode of so-called business meetings was over.

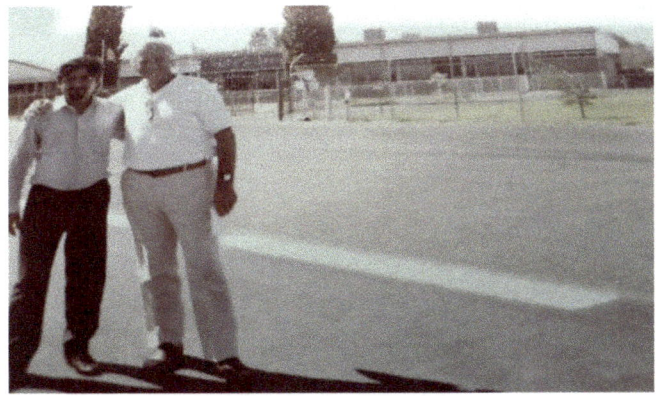

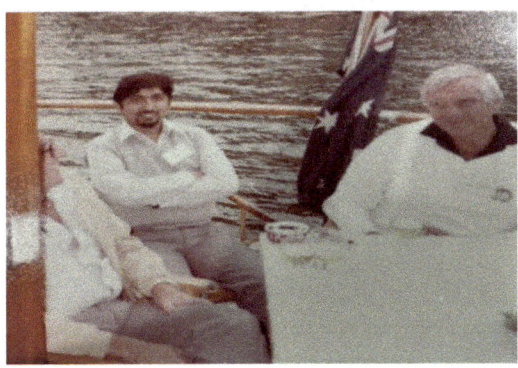

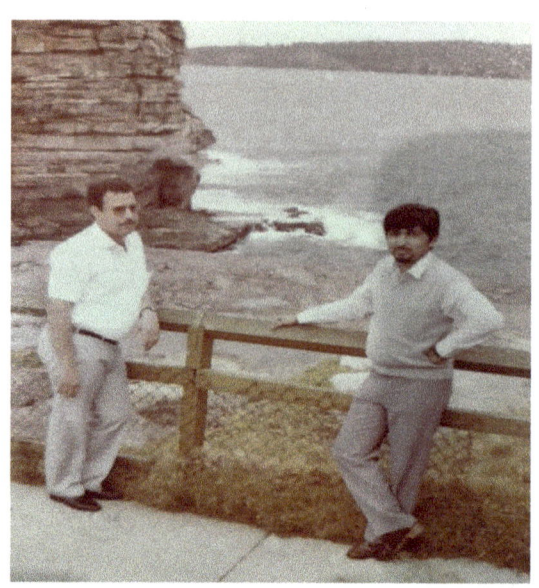

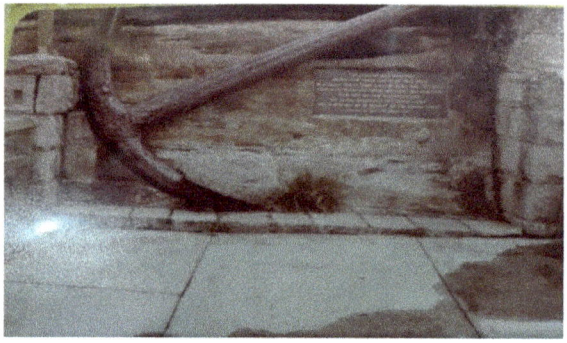

Glimpses of Australia

Next day we were supposed to visit the mining areas, at Gove, an island for bauxite mining and its shipping protocols. My company in Saudi Arabia required, 40,000 MT every quarter. We boarded a six-seater plane and landed on a red air strip. In the name of airport there was mere a log cabin. Exiting the gate, I saw another log cabin with board atop, depicting idli, dosa, vada and like and Malayalam script beneath. I looked at the General Manager, Marketing in utter surprise. He innocently asked, if I didn't know that when Armstrong, first landed on moon, heard 'illay poun'. I understood Keralites were so enterprising could be found anywhere. Further ahead were dwellings of ab-origin, naked, drunk and intoxicated. We mounted a jeep and drove through dense forests to NABALCO Plant for the manufacturing of Aluminum. It was state-of- the art facility. Slag generated were discharged into a huge pit of 500X500X5 meters. I was fascinated and asked if a sample of this waste could be analyzed for aluminum content in their laboratory. A composite sample was sent to the laboratory. Then we moved to the mining area and saw the longest conveyor belt, 19.5 km from mines to the shipping yard through dense forest. Upon return analytical report was ready. It depicted 48% of aluminum content. Something flashed into my mind and asked what will be fate of this huge quantity of the waste. They said, it was their major dilemma. I asked how much it would cost if we bought. They said free and were thankful. We made a deal to transport this waste to our plant in Saudi Arabia. This proved to be my first ever Recycling project, saving millions of dollars for the company.

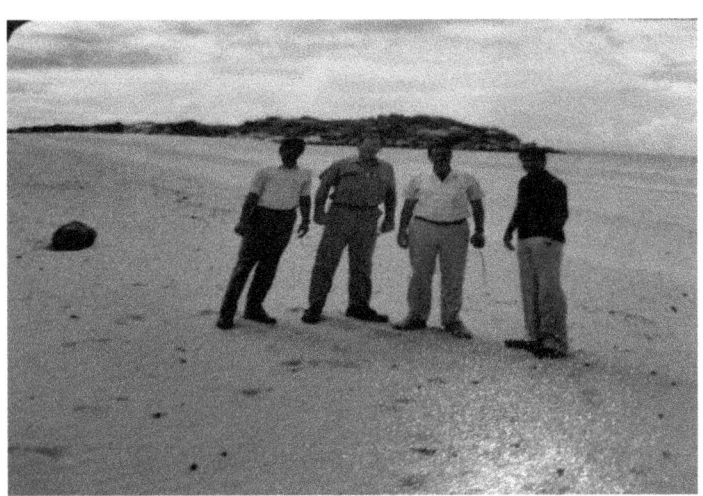

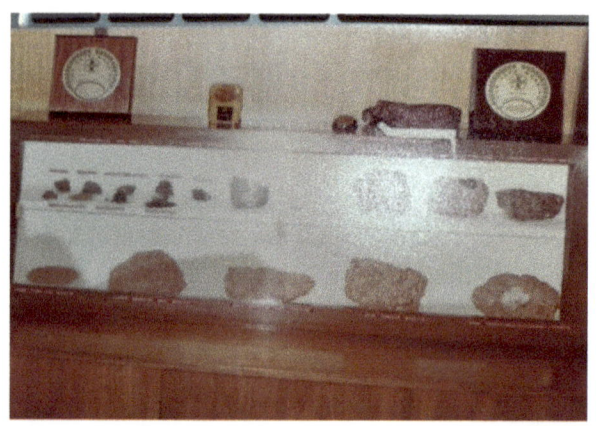
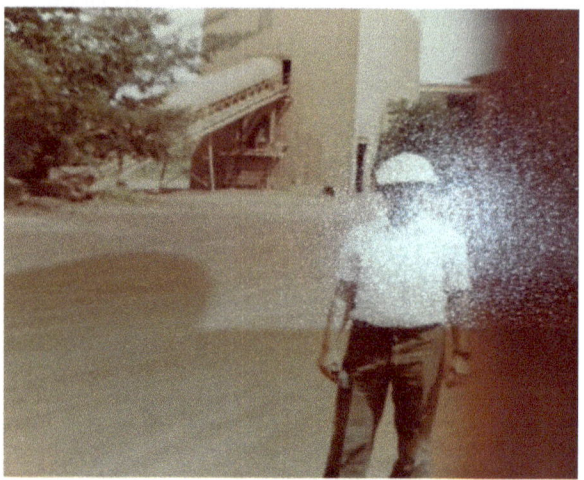
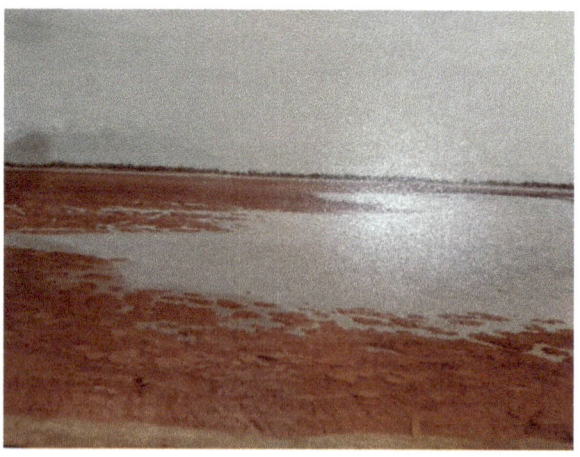

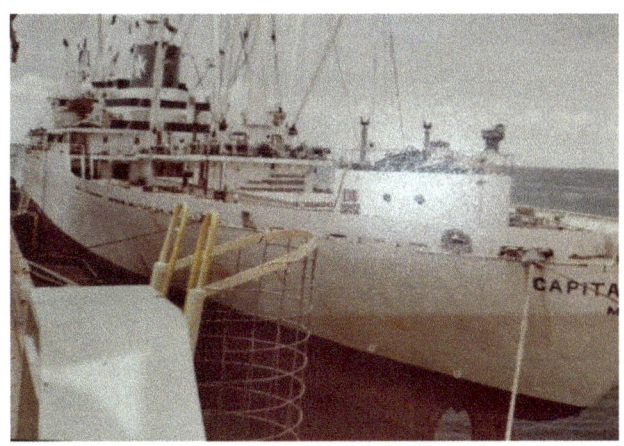

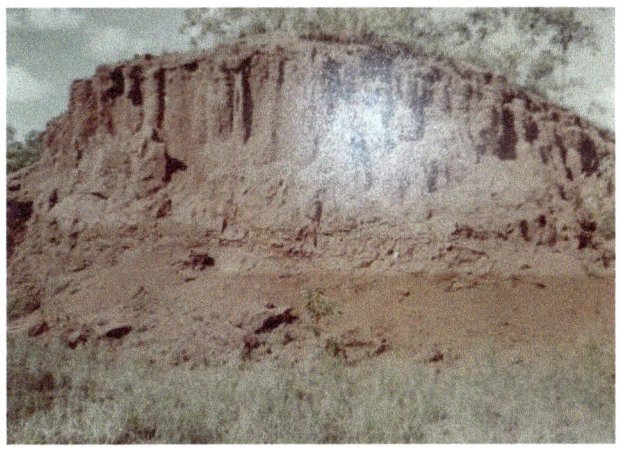

Glimpses of NABALCO, GOVE

We travelled to Darwin, Townsville, Alice Spring and finally Sydney. Spectacular experience enroute showcasing opals, aborigin art and craft and a lot more. After couple of months, completing Quality Report and signing of the Supply Agreement returned back to the base. First time came to know what 'Night life' meant and what wife swapping was.

Upon return it was due date of our third's arrival in this world, Athar. It was such a joy for not only us but the entire family camp. Amazing experience of Arab ladies who used to bring loads of

Arabian cuisine, their care for mother and the baby, including diaper change, were unforgettable Arab hospitality experience.

A couple of weeks later, I was again given task of a team leader to lead chemists for specific analytical protocols' training at the research facility of **KRUPP POLYSIUS**, Neubeckum, Germany and for me to get the Laboratory Management exposure.

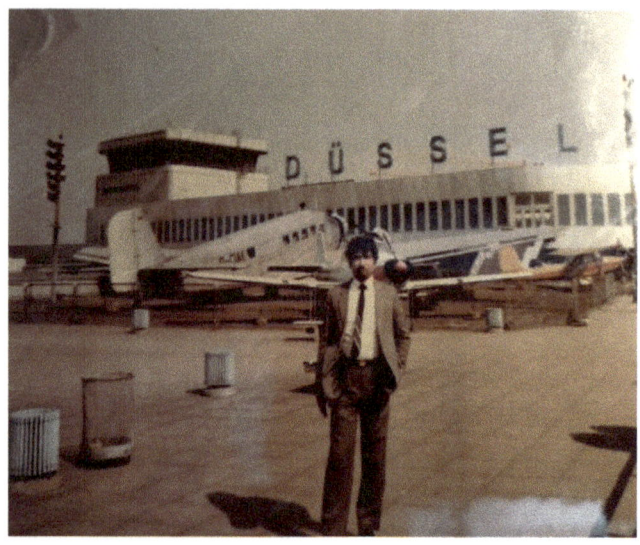

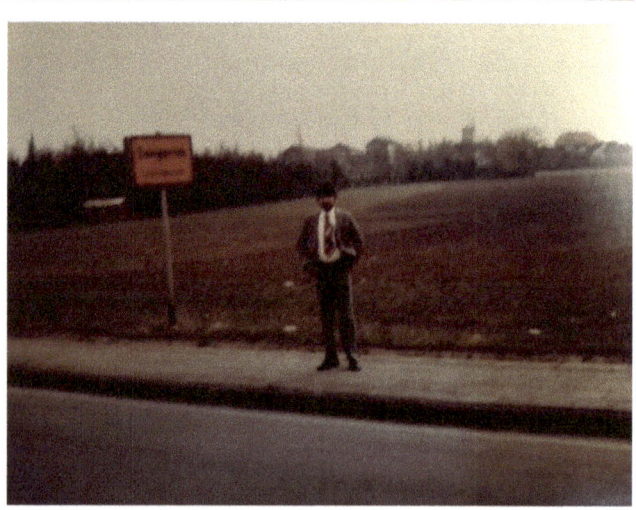

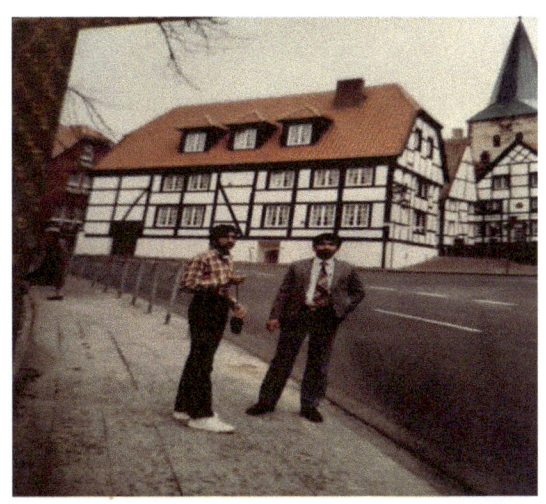
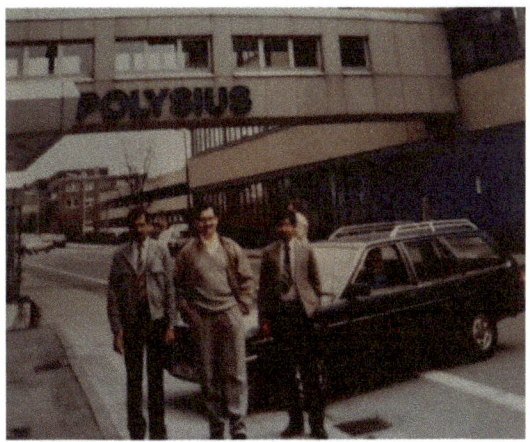
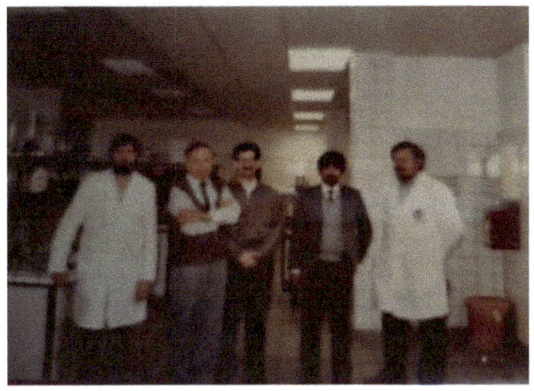

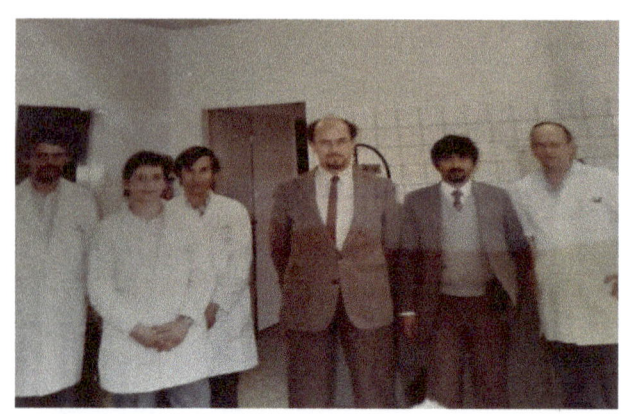

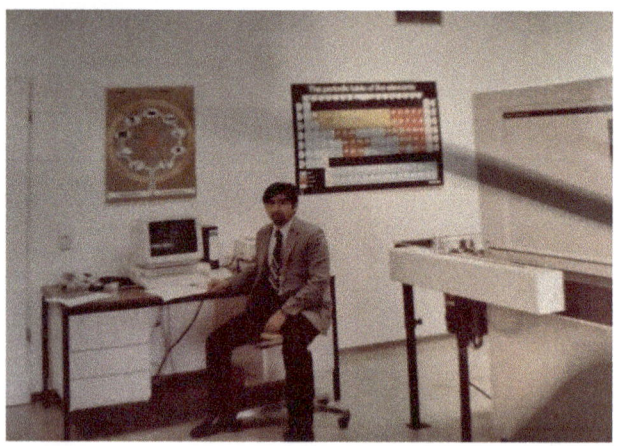

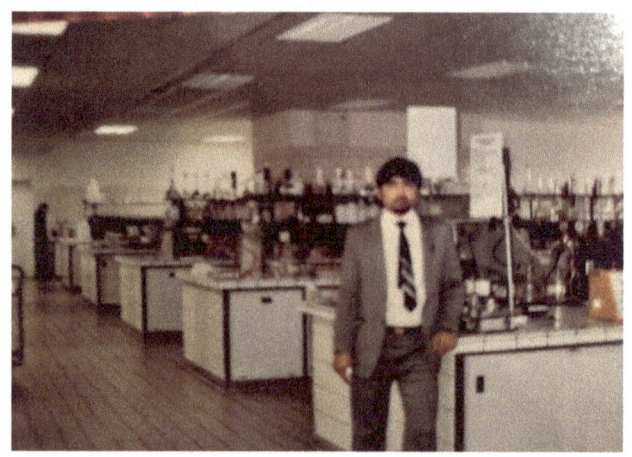

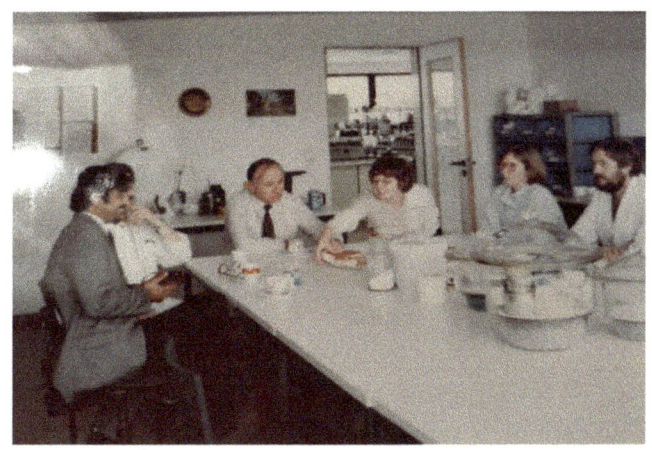

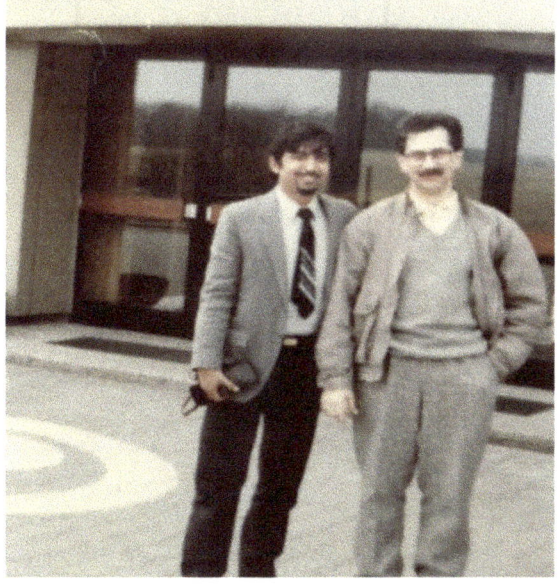

Glimpses of Polysius Neubekum

On the next weekend taken a train to Paris and visited all its attractions on a tourist bus. Included in the ticket was at the end, a live show with champagne. I asked the waiter if soft drink could be served instead of champagne. He was so delighted and said would take himself and served 7UP throughout the show.

I left Paris via Belgium back to Germany. When my passport was checked, I was told to follow and came to know, I needed transit visa for Belgium.

Next weekend flew aboard British Airways to Heathrow, London to meet my cousin brother and his family at Greenford, Middlesex. He showed all London attractions including famed Oxford University which was an inspiration for Sir Syed Ahmad Khan for making the AMU.

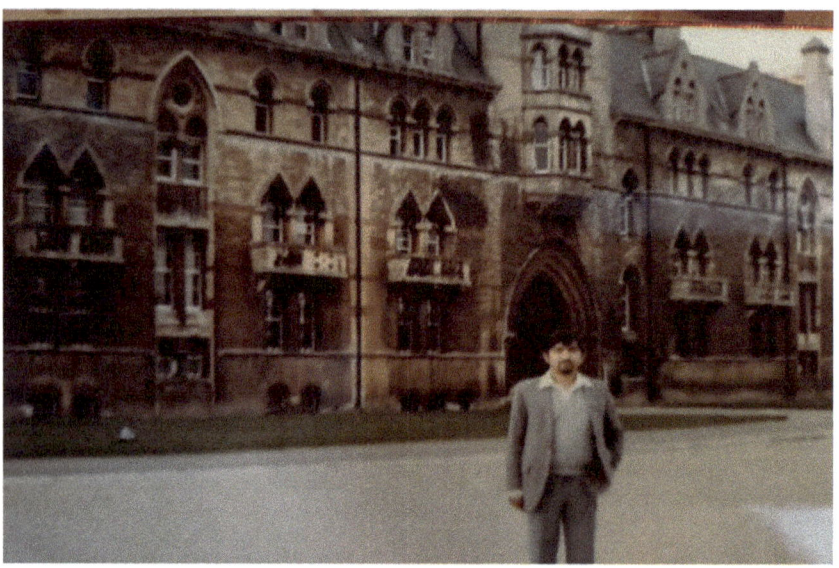

The following weekend I visited Munster, city of university, Dusseldorf, Hem, and their impressive country side.

Our assignment concluded and we boarded Lufthansa for Dammam. We had a stopover at Frankfurt for a couple of hours and was exposed at the airport with Sex Toys. I saw a few of smart Indian looking girls and boys. I introduced myself. They were in fact Saudis speaking flawless English. While interacting, came to know, they were in the USA on Saudi Scholarship. One of them informed they were privileged students. When they landed, were housed in a villa each with a teenager girl to teach American etiquettes of speaking, interacting, eating, drinking and ultimately to bedroom performances. These kids were more American than American themselves.

We returned back loaded with knowledge and diversified experience. Gradually I became quite disappointed with my job. It became day in and day out just supervising 94 staff and signing papers and attending meetings. There was nothing like value addition in my work or any charm. Further higher positions in the industry were in the hands of majority community of India, Egypt and Pakistan. Our Indian counterparts used to play Indian politics there as well. Further schooling for Saima and Ahmad became a nightmare. I could see disgust in their eyes but they never complained. They were not growing normally. I took the hard decision to quit my job and return back to India. I put them in school and started scouting for job back in Saudi Arabia. Fortunately, I got a break at the AMU as Lecturer in the Department of Applied Chemistry, ZHCOET, my dream job to teach at the AMU.

Life was very much content. I was given a task to establish an Environmental Laboratory at AMU Women's College and take classes of Home Science of Second Year BSc. I also started guiding couple of PhD aspirants in Environmental Chemistry. On professional front I was very much satisfied until my son Ahmad had to be admitted at the JNMC for appendicitis pains. He was to be operated. I was given a list of items to be brought for the operation from outside. It was almost the end of the month when my financial situation used to be on red alert. I had to run pillar to post to get just a thousand rupee. That day decided to go back to Saudi Arabia.

A week later I received a call from Jubail Industrial City for an interview the following day. Interview by an American had been quite heartening. I was supposed to establish an Environmental

Management Facility with an Environmental Laboratory. I was selected for the job. Some of my teaching colleague who were not yet confirmed, were relieved but my students were sad. I resigned and left for my new work place.

My company, National Environmental Preservation Co. (BeeA'h) was supposed to treat and dispose Hazardous Wastes emanating from petroleum refining, petrochemical and chemical industries. It was an ardent task for me to conceptualize and do the needful. I had to learn, so used to go to the KFUPM's library through friends.

Within six months almost, prepared basic conceptual design of the Hazardous Waste Management Facility (HWMF), comprising of Class I and Class II Landfills, an Evaporation Pond with Sprinkler System, an Environmental Laboratory, Sludge Bunkers, Curbed Concrete Pad (CCP) with Catchment Pit, Porta Site Offices and Conference Room, Weighbridge and Guard house, Car Park, Open Drum and Bulk Storage, Shaded Drum Storage, Firefighting Systems. We commissioned the facility and started operation of the facility. I had to be involved with the Marketing Head for the business development. We participated in the national and internation conferences, presenting papers, lecturing university staff and administration, putting articles in the leading papers newspapers, magazines and visiting senior staff of industries and speaking from their perspective. I became a star environmental mentor for all those staff who were unaware of nuances associated with the Hazardous Waste management in particular and Environmental Management in general.

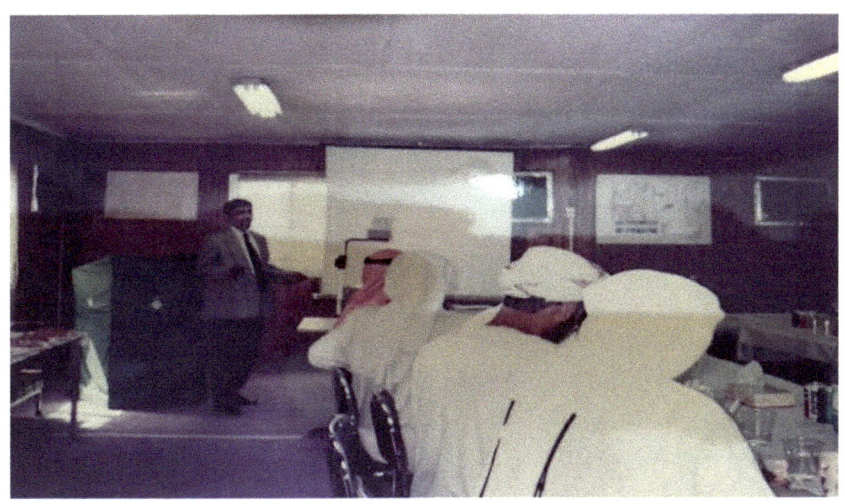

Business started pouring in millions of dollars' worth. Capital investment of 12.5 million Saudi Riyals were returned to the investors with 5% profit and balance profit was used for the upgrade of the facility and the environmental laboratory. My understanding and interest in the field grew over the time and added Environmental Monitoring, Environmental Analysis, Environmental Consultancy, Contaminated Site Remediation etc. to our profile. We spread our wings beyond the Jubail Industrial City covering Ras Tanura Aramco petroleum refining, Dammam chemical industries, Dhahran Aramco, Riyadh chemical industries, Yanbu Sabic and Aramco etc. The company made millions of Riyals. Need was felt to add thermal treatment facility as well. But what, First Gulf War had erupted. Being the Facility Manager, I was 24X7 on duties. People were fleeing Kuwait and entering Saudi Arabia in masses. They had been taken care by Saudi Arabia to house them and feed them appropriately per their Master's dictate. As people, Kuwaiti were the worst I had ever encountered, full of pseudo-pride and ill- mannered despite what had befallen upon them.

An agreement for the war waste management was signed between the Allied Forces and my company. I had to drive almost daily to Kuwait borders which was under US Armed forces' control, to coordinate shipment of waste to our HWMF. It was mere a coincidence that my family had gone to India on winter break. I eye-witnessed, Iraqi scud being intercepted by US Patriots. One of the scud missiles, was intercepted right above my roof top and the impact was so great that my apartment was badly damaged.

As the Facility Manager, I was supposed to prepare the Emergency Contingency Plan to safeguard people working under me. I could smell unrest in my people. They were secretly planning to take company vehicles to run to the safety. I went to the General Manager, Saad I. Al-Inaizi, and expressed my views in the Head Office some 20 km away, comparatively at a safer location. Instead of understanding my concerns, he said you Indians are cowards. My upper section simply got blown off and I snapped back, if you were brave, would not have called nanny forces to protect you despite it was not your war and to become their stooge and left his office to do what was appropriate to be done. I had to spend most nights, awake near the facility in my car watching sky on fire from a distance and keeping an eye on my facility. I had to just take naps at road side to catch up with my sleep. I had hurt my boss's ego. He did all he could to intimidate me.

Iraq was bombed from all sides by Allied Forces and Saudi Arabian forces with Gulf alliance forces. Even Saudis were running desperately out of war region towards Jeddah, Makkah and Madina. Media criminals had painted such a picture of WMD in their domain to spread fear and hate for Saddam Hussain, as world would come to come to an end soon. In the name of WMD pretext, carpet bombing begun with full media coverage as if film shooting was in progress. Media even covered things that really never had happened. Saudis were so much brain washed that they became as ruthless as Americans to topple down Saddam regime and serve US ambitions in the region. Saudi media were not behind, CNN, BBC etc. in propaganda machinery to support US interests in the region to the extent to paint the crises to the Holy War. Those who were think tanks for the interest of the region, fearing chaos in the Muslim World, were simply silenced, put behind bars or even eradicated. A few incidences, witnessed are mere the tip of the iceberg.

Top US and Allied Forces personnel had been housed in SWCC Residential Areas because they were having world class facilities. It was Ramadan, at a manager's place people were invited for breaking fast. A lady major was on the street to the swimming pool in bikinis. The Manager came out and requested the Major, sister it is Ramadan, please be in modest dresses on the street as we are very conscious of our tradition. The Major called someone and in minutes Saudi Security Forces appeared and dragged the Manager holding his beards to their darkened van, shouting how dare he could insult their guest. The Manager disappeared simply, never to be seen again.

People were jailed and many were put in Empty Quarters from where none could return and a lot many were simply executed.

No white skinned were ever checked on check points while non-Americans, non-Europeans, even the Saudis with beard and in their traditional outfit were rudely grilled by Saudi Security Forces.

The Imams who raised their voices against, were dragged out of mosques to oblivion.

A shipload of girls was brought to the port. Only Saudi youth were allowed to enter and enjoy free of cost with dine and wine.

Pornographic magazines were rampantly distributed to Saudis in particular to rejoice American and European culture.

Cultural invasion had begun!

After destruction of Iraq, its heritage, its economy and the might in the region, we were given a multi-million-dollar contract, to clear up the so -called war mess. The mess included the first and second World Wars' chemicals and war utensils for disposal besides new stuff to dispose of on the Saudi Soil and with Saudi Money. Hazardous waste treatment and disposal remains most expensive affair in the USA and Europe. Gulf War cover, conveniently made Saudi Arabia a dumping site for their so-called friends and that too on Saudi Arabia's cost.

We made millions of dollars, through waste management, sales of goods, reuse of stuff.

During demobilization we were contracted to even clear up camps, in the name of municipal waste. Our workers got appliances, practically new, cameras and things like that, including dollar bills. Truckloads of pornographic literature and magazines were disposed in the Sanitary landfills.

During the war period, I had been given responsibility to be local support to our US Associate, Environmental Technology, San Florida, for the installation of a Pilot Wastewater Treatment Plant at Ar- Razi, a Sabic affiliate. It was for the treatment of wastewater (effluent) in order to recycle them in their process and be able to zero discharge in the gulf.

I drove CEO and three Vice Presidents in 3-piece suits, to the project site to start their deliberations. They did what was supposed to be done. When they started the plant, they seemed perplexed. First the jackets were removed, tie was loosened, sleeves were then folded. I asked them if I could be of some help. They seemed relieved. My Dr prefix had earlier also been respected those days. I went to my laboratory and made a few experiments. I returned to the project site and changed set points. The plant started running as it was designed. They were very much delighted for the success of the project. Wemhoff, the CEO, wrote a detailed Letter of Appreciation to my boss, describing my contribution to the project. For the first time my boss's attitude towards me was changed and got first ever increment in my remunerations. Wemhoff offered even a job of the Vice President in his organization, almost three times remuneration. I refused politely as I was satisfied with my job and there was a balance in my family life and professional life, between deen (Spiritual) and duniya (material). He was surprised to find, an Indian refusing such a lucrative offer.

I had completed several multi-million Riyals projects very successfully and presented several papers in various International Conferences.

White skin color being Saudi's weakness, one New Zealander and a British were hired as Engineering Services and Business Development Managers respectively. I was supposed to give them orientation of the business.

After three months I was given a letter to report to the Engineering Services Manager. It was a literal shock but could not resign due to family circumstances.

I started reporting as had been directed. After a few months, I was called upon by the top gun for telling me that my performance was not up to the mark. I said it would take 45 minutes to respond.

I drove back to my office and took all my files to him depicting my deliberation to that date. It was revealed that the New Zealander used to change my cover letter with his and submit. Saudi ego did not allow the top gun to be even regretful. I had decided to resign at an appropriate time.

The day my elder children appeared for the last examination of the High School; I submitted my resignation with an advance 3-months' notice. During the notice period I presented a paper in an International Conference in Dubai. My paper was considered the best . Uninformed, MTV was taking my live interview and it was watched by top executive of ADNOC Abu Dhabi. Next morning I received a call from him asking if I was interested in joining ADNOC. I affirmed. After completion of my notice period, I joined ADNOC but got bored soon. Office environment was not what I was used to, it used to be a gossip factory. Further I was supposed to report to a person who came to ADNOC through sports category and got promoted over a period of time. He could not either write or speak English. Further all my deliberations were supposed to be only signed by him as per protocol without my mention. Terms and conditions of employment had been quite lucrative but I started getting disinterested in work and resigned within the probation period. My only contribution to ADNOC had been when I joined, they were having one Environmental Engineer per refinery and after I left, they had Environmental Directorate. My proposal was accepted but not in my name or to my credit.

When I was about to leave Abu Dhabi, received a call from Saudi Company for Environmental Works which was in infancy. I was offered position of the Technical Manager cum Deputy General Manager.

I started my new assignment with great enthusiasm. Developed their facility and prepared their Systems and Protocols and bagged several projects and represented them in an international conference with my latest paper.

I realized that they were bad pay masters. Never salary was given on time and that too not without insistence to pay. I got really vexed by the close of the year and resigned and left for my hometown in India.

Sooner, I landed in Delhi, I received a call from the United Medical Group who offered me a job as Manager Environmental Affairs on a better package. I joined them on first of Ramadan. I was housed in the Holiday Inn for a month. They were catering to the needs of the Ministry of Health and Defense. I was given a lavish office and a family accommodation in a Western Compound with all amenities; Olympian swimming pool, Gym, Recreation Room etc. with all hard furnishings. This year I cleared Registered Environmental Manager (REM) examination from the National Registry of Environmental Professionals, Illinois. I was featured by the Saudi Gazette.

Within a year, I got uneasy to find they were nothing but brokers. A million-dollar Environmental System used to be sold for 10 million USD by bribing a million.

I resigned and joined Abdullah Hashim Group (AHG) to develop their Environmental Division as the Manager Environmental Division, in their Head Quarters based in Jeddah. It was the best period of my life due to proximity with Makkah and Madinah. Every day we used to pray Maghrib and Isha in Haram of Makkah and on weekends used to visit Madinah. Just before the close of the year, due to Pakistani politics, I received a letter telling, that due to the non-feasibility of the project, the division is being closed down. It was a disheartening experience.

Due to family situation, I had to do something and did. I joined BeeA'H again as an Environmental and Business Development Consultant. Within a year I established their FEMS and Stack Testing Section.

Now a high-profile professional was not required and I was without a job with a family of five children to feed and educate. I joined Al-Jabr Group, as the General Manager but on a salary, half of the previous one. In six months, Systems and Protocols were developed, licenses achieved, I became redundant.

Then there came a mega project and SEW requested me to join for preparation of their proposal and head the project. Having no option handy, I rejoined them back. We got the project. My CEO did not listen to my advice for International Project

Management. As a result, the project was taken back and given over night to another company. I became redundant again.

I joined ENDEV, Jeddah. Here the GM was a fanatic. Wanted projects without meeting project requirements. I had heated conversation with him and lost the job within six months.

Soon after joined GEMS, Jeddah as an Environmental Specialist. Due to South Indian mafia and Saudi unprofessional politics, I had to leave within two months leaving behind my household worth lakhs there to join Haif Group in the Eastern Province to look after their environmental monitoring projects. Got them ISO-9001 and ISO-14001 certified but soon the company was sold out.

I then joined Saudi Arkan to establish their Environmental Business in the Eastern Province. Conceptual Design to permitting to Systems and Protocols development etc. were achieved in a year besides signing MOUs with several international outfits to establish business on a sound footing. As I was still fighting my legal battle with the SEW, was not in a position to travel abroad and so both GM and the CEO were supposed to, but they did not due to language barrier, I suppose... This antagonized the International Joint Venture partners. I was told to conclude my assignment and leave.

Fortunately, soon got another good break and joined Our Green Environment as the General Manager cum President's Consultant. As the company was mere on the paper, prepared the blue print, systems and protocols, documents for permits, land allocation, SIDF loans etc. However, due to lack of funds, the project slowed down to a standstill. I had to once again pack my baggage. My legal battle concluded with a tragedy of corruption. SEW bribed heavily to the document control in-charge and got documents changed. They also did buy out my lawyer in the last hearing. He did not turn up. As a result, despite I won the battle on paper, lost all my money worth a million dollar. I left for India and started taking up mini assignments.

In 2015, one of my trainees called me up and wanted me to join a budding outfit MESCO in the JIS, Eastern Province, where he was the President. Here too, the same exercise was carried out leading to SIDF Loans, ISO-14001 and OHSAS Certifications, signing of several MOUs with French, German, Spanish, Polish, US and UK based outfits for the technology transfer. When the investment arrived, some 30 million SAR. The CEO managed to get transferred funds to his personal account and bought a luxurious villa, Rolls Royce etc. As a result, could not make payments to contractors and sub-contractors. They stopped the construction works for the installation and commissioning of treatment systems, expected from abroad. The company collapsed, so did I. I returned home in 2017. In 2019, I got another project and started working on it for a couple of months and pandemic of corona engulfed the world and businesses. I managed to return home losing all my money. Then I was victim of Covid followed by by-pass surgery. I became vegetable. In late 2023, one of my junior staff, a Jordanian insisted to come and join hands with him for the Gulf Elite establishment. I felt was once again alive, probably due to proximity with Makkah and Madina. In just three months, I established the company and got several projects. However, the Jordanian and myself were on different wavelengths of understanding. He wanted to mint money by dumping and me as per national and international protocols. Result was, I had to leave in order to avoid professional prostitution.

CHAPTER 6

Journey from Environmental Scientist to Environmemntal Writer

Although I wrote Research Papers and Articles during PhD program, wrote articles for the leading newspapers, presented papers on the national and the international conferences; my struggle for the BALANCE continued and wrote my first book, Balance, an essence of my professional journey to date, which has been published recently. Now I am venturing on MIRAGE, my autobiography.

Several books on Environmental Management are in the pipeline while continuing my International Consultancy Services.

CHAPTER 7

Chronic Consequences of Shizophrenia

My greatest setback in life throughout, had been borrowing from my friends in order to keeping my generosity to people around me and sometimes for keeping my boat afloat.

Qarz ki petay thay mai lekin samajhtay thay ki han,

Rang layegi hamari faqa masti ek din

(used to take wine by borrowing and used to think, that one day this rejoicing in hunger would reflect)

In my student life, particularly, my friend who recently retired as a professor, Dr. Ghulam Mursaleen, who had given me his signed check book, to withdraw as and when required. I was only able to return when I was on my first job in Saudi Arabia. I never ever met a person like him in my life. He was and is so sweet, never ever put my dignity on stake. My heartfelt appreciation and gratefulness belong to him.

Another, friend and a classmate, Dr. Suhail Ahmad Ansari had been my savior throughout my turbulent professional career. He unfailingly used to be on my side when owns didn't bother about me, whether I was right or wrong.

Two Pakistani adored me very much. Iqbal Ahmad Chaudhry, then the General Manager of Olayan-Descon, Jubail, Saudi Arabia gave me a loan of over a crore over a period of time for various of my overtures of supporting family and friends and genuinely deserving. I could pay back, years after. Ijaz Ahmad Rabbani used to send in lakhs during my joblessness and lockdown when everyone used to shy away.

Retired Professor of Pharmacology, Dr. Iqtedar H Zaidi proved to be another savior during two testing hours.

There were others too.

My second major weakness had been, blind trust in people and had paid heavily in that account, yet do not regret.

My WhatsApp /Messenger/Facebook friendships with opposite gender, across the globe had been my third consequence of Schizophrenia. I simply enjoyed it without any evil intention whatsoever. I liked to emotionally massage tormented ladies across continents making them feel better. Some accepted Islam as well. My friendship led to some conversions in Europe too. Some of them even played dirty upon my refusal to be with them forever. Some even morphed my pics and put on the internet causing a lot of embarrassment. A lot of them did propose, and I had to stop communications with many.

Another consequence had been my carelessness for valuables and lost hundreds of thousands in France, Spain and elsewhere by pick pocketers and others.

CHAPTER 8

Confession of Being Schizophrenic

I have made several mistakes in life, mostly circumstantial, some due to being impulsive at times and some due to ignorance.

Most mistakes had been committed post departure of my wife from this world. I was myself imbalanced and was supposed to be a balancing force.

I should have not married at all after Farro. I had been looking for something impossible, keeping my mother's example in mind.

I was looking for a mother, which was later realized, was next to impossible. My three adventures did prove that.

If at all, I had to marry, should have married to someone not married before and among those who did not have children and longed to have.

All these years I had to endure comparison with Exes on grounds not decent to describe. The subd widowed)sequent marriages did not serve my purpose at all rather aggravated my problems. No one could prove to be mothers. They were mothers of their own begotten children and my false notion of complying with Sunnah (marrying divorced and widowed) proved to be erroneous. Whether religious or ultra- modern, all proved to be only materialistic, at the end of the exercise.

I should not have been emotionally charged for my children post their mother's departure, and should have left the matter to the God to resolve the dilemma. I feel responsible for spoiling Omar in particular. I should have left both Omar and Sarah on God's resolution. Also, should have not considered Saima and Ahmad matured enough to influence my conviction. They were then, incapable of handling affairs despite they did their best from their perspectives. They were basically representing me, in my absence, but that proved to be counter-productive for all at the end.

CHAPTER 9

Epilogue

دیکھتے کرم اہل تماشائے ؔغالب بھیس ہم کا فقیروں کر بنا
غالب مرزا ہیں

(Bana kar faqeeroun ka hum bhes Ghalib, Tamashaye ahl e karam dekhtay hai

(In of a popper, I watch grand show of generous).

When I visit a doctor, he/she hardly is concerned about the patient's ailment but only in fees and tests and wants you to speak yourself in seconds as next patient is waiting (PRIVATE PRACTIONERS), if you happen to be with doctors in institutes, they talk like administrators hardly raising their heads to have personal perception.

Psychiatry and Behavioral Science have different concept in my dear city Aligarh.

One well known doctor without checking prescribed medication or doing anything, prescribes medicines and concludes something on no basis.

Duniya (meray ghar ki duniya) samjhay mujhko pagal,

Mayn sumjhoun duniya ko pagal.

(People think I am an insane, I feel they are insane).

I leave it to readers and true professionals to infer whether the case is of schizophrenia?

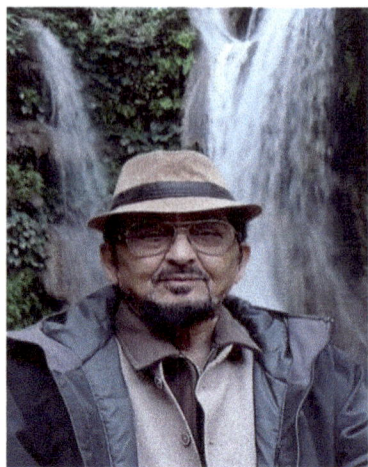

References/ Publications

1. Schizophrenia - Symptoms and causes - Mayo Clinic
2. Balance (Mezan), ISBN:978-93-6249-604-1, 2024
3. Mirage, ISBN:978-93-6249-285-2, 2025
4. Hazard is My Trade, 2025 (In press)
5. 'Selecting the best waste management technologies (treatment & disposal) for industrial non-hazardous, industrial hazardous and medical wastes', Sulaiman, Afsar M., Waste Expo, Dubai, 1996
6. "Jubail a model of environmental ethics", Sulaiman, Afsar M., Special Report, Saudi Gazette, 29 October 1994,
7. "Hazard is Their Trade", Sulaiman, Afsar M. Panorama. Saudi Gazette, 02 February 1995
8. "Case Study – Operation of the Beea'h Hazardous Waste Facility", Sulaiman, Afsar M., 3rd Annual Middle East Convention, Waste Management and Waste Minimization, Dubai, 22-25 April 1995
9. Cost Effective Management of Oily Wastes, Sulaiman, Afsar M. Second Specialty Conference on Environmental Progress in the Petroleum & Petrochemical Industries, Bahrain, Proceedings, OW-87, P413-425, November 17-19, 1997
10. "The Enormous Task of Managing Medical Waste", Sulaiman Afsar M., Nation, Special Report, Saudi Gazette, 03 May 1998
11. "Present Scenario, Tomorrow's Vision, Hazardous Waste Management", Sulaiman, Afsar M., Editorial Page, Comments, Saudi Gazette, 08 May 1998
12. "Cement Kiln as waste treatment and energy recovery option", Sulaiman, Afsar M. Panorama, Science, Saudi Gazette, 10 August 1998

13. Status of Environmental Activities in Saudi Arabia, Sulaiman Afsar M., Saudi Gazette, World Environment Day Supplement, June 2001

14. "Cost Effective Management of Spent Catalyst from Hydrocarbon Processing Industries", Sulaiman, Afsar M., Middle East, Petrotech 96" Conference, Bahrain 10-12 June 1996

About the Author

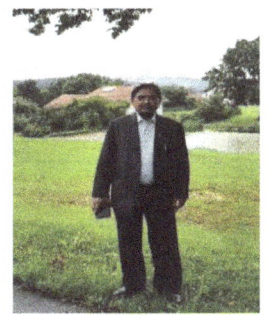

Dr. Afsar M. Sulaiman, a Qualified Environmental Professional (QEP) from Pittsburgh, Registered Environmental Manager from Illinois, Environmental Scientist and an International Consultant, has recently published his books, Balance and Mirage and now publishing an essence of his professional journey expanding to almost four decades. The new book, HAZARD is my trade, which is practically a hand book, meant for Environmental Science and Engineering students, teachers and professionals.

He is an Alig who was enrolled in 1972 in PUC and completed his PhD in Environmental Chemistry in 1983 from the Department of Applied Chemistry, Z. H. College of Engineering & Technology, AMU, Aligarh. His career started from the IIT Bombay as a Research Scientist. He was responsible for the establishment of the first Environmental Management Company in the Middle East, National Environmental Preservation Co. Jubail, Saudi Arabia. During his four decades of services for environmental cause, he was awarded International Man of the Year was featured in Five Hundred Leaders of Influence, MARQUIS Who's Who in the World, Saudi Gazette in 1998-99. He presented his papers in several international conferences. He travelled the world to find the best environmental technologies, best suited for the Middle East in general and Saudi Arabia in particular. He has established several environmental companies, outfits and establishments across Saudi Arabia, Bahrain, Qatar and UAE

www.ingramcontent.com/pod-product-compliance
Lightning Source LLC
LaVergne TN
LVHW061626070526
838199LV00070B/6594